My Ultimate Dash Diet Plan

50 Easy and Balanced Recipes for Your Health

Eleonore Barlow

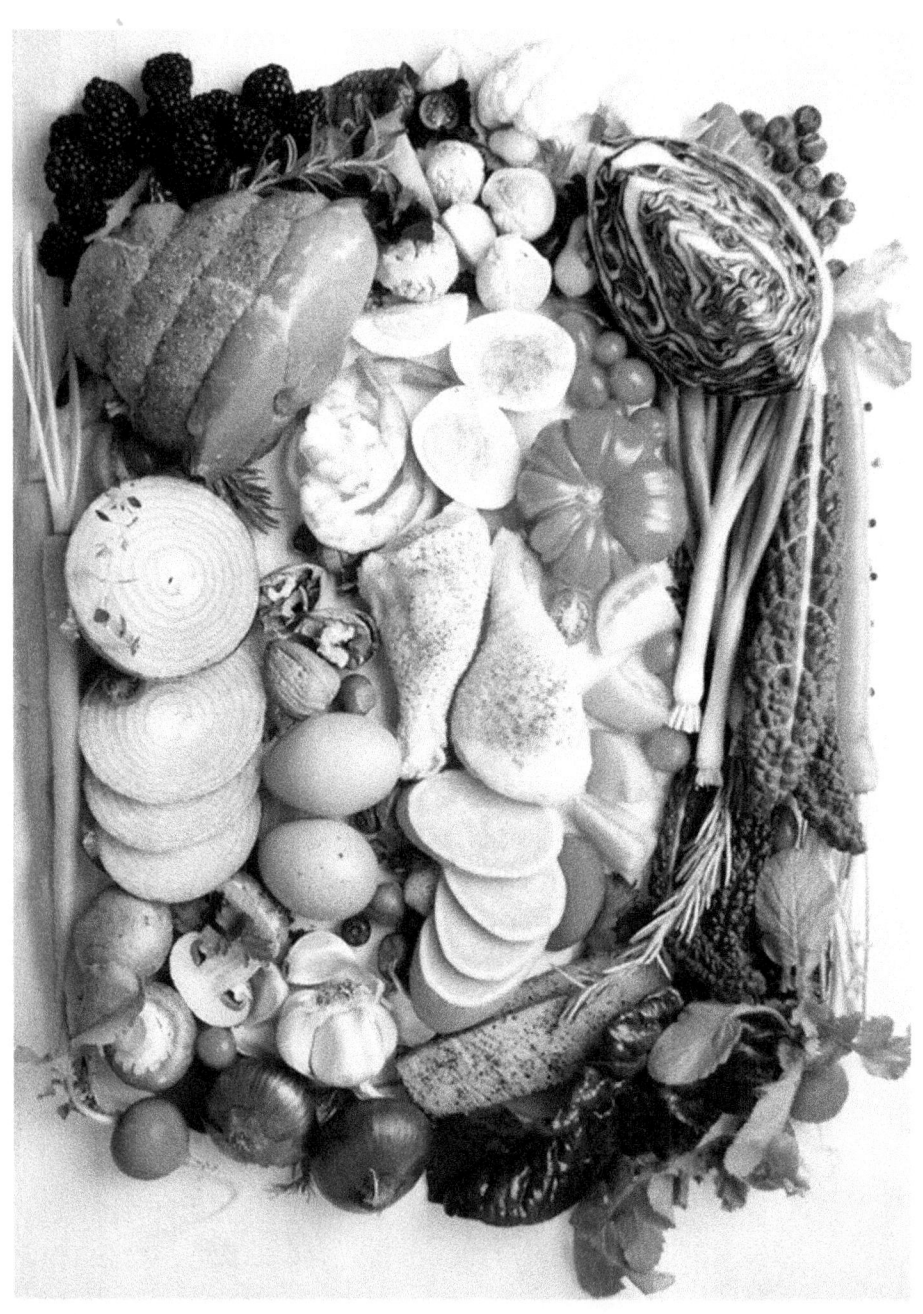

© Copyright 2021 - All rights reserved.

The content contained within this book may not be reproduced, duplicated or transmitted without direct written permission from the author or the publisher.
Under no circumstances will any blame or legal responsibility be held against the publisher, or author, for any damages, reparation, or monetary loss due to the information contained within this book. Either directly or indirectly.

Legal Notice:
This book is copyright protected. This book is only for personal use. You cannot amend, distribute, sell, use, quote or paraphrase any part, or the content within this book, without the consent of the author or publisher.

Disclaimer Notice:
Please note the information contained within this document is for educational and entertainment purposes only. All effort has been executed to present accurate, up to date, and reliable, complete information. No warranties of any kind are declared or implied. Readers acknowledge that the author is not engaging in the rendering of legal, financial, medical or professional advice. The content within this book has been derived from various sources. Please consult a licensed professional before attempting any techniques outlined in this book.
By reading this document, the reader agrees that under no circumstances is the author responsible for any losses, direct or indirect, which are incurred as a result of the use of information contained within this document, including, but not limited to, — errors, omissions, or inaccuracies.

Table of Contents

- FUDGE BROWNIES ... 6
- POMEGRANATE QUINOA PORRIDGE ... 8
- STEWED APPLES ... 10
- CINNAMON AND COCONUT PORRIDGE ... 11
- COCONUT PORRIDGE ... 13
- CINNAMON PEAR OATMEAL ... 15
- BANANA AND WALNUT BOWL ... 17
- SCRAMBLED PESTO EGGS ... 19
- BARLEY PORRIDGE ... 21
- MUSTARD CHICKEN ... 23
- CHICKEN AND CARROT STEW ... 25
- THE DELISH TURKEY WRAP ... 27
- ALMOND BUTTERNUT CHICKEN ... 29
- ZUCCHINI ZOODLES WITH CHICKEN AND BASIL ... 31
- BEEF SOUP ... 33
- AMAZING GRILLED CHICKEN AND BLUEBERRY SALAD ... 35
- CLEAN CHICKEN AND MUSHROOM STEW ... 38
- ELEGANT PUMPKIN CHILI DISH ... 40
- SIMPLE GARLIC AND LEMON SOUP ... 42
- HEALTHY CUCUMBER SOUP ... 44
- MUSHROOM CREAM SOUP ... 46
- CURIOUS ROASTED GARLIC SOUP ... 48
- AMAZING ROASTED CARROT SOUP ... 50
- SIMPLE PUMPKIN SOUP ... 52
- COCONUT AVOCADO SOUP ... 54
- COCONUT ARUGULA SOUP ... 56
- AWESOME CABBAGE SOUP ... 58
- BAKED ZUCCHINI WRAPPED FISH ... 60

HEART-WARMING MEDI TILAPIA	62
BAKED SALMON AND ORANGE JUICE	64
LEMON AND ALMOND BUTTER COD	67
SHRIMP SCAMPI	69
LIGHT BEEF CHILI	71
INSALATA GRECA	74
CRUDITIES	77
HERRING WITH ONIONS	78
SIMPLE GINGERBREAD MUFFINS	79
FANTASTIC CAULIFLOWER BAGELS	81
NUTMEG NOUGATS	83
LIMEY SAVORY PIE	85
SUPREME RASPBERRY CHOCOLATE BOMBS	87
THE PERFECT ORANGE PONZU	90
HEARTY CASHEW AND ALMOND BUTTER	92
REFRESHING MANGO AND PEAR SMOOTHIE	94
EPIC PINEAPPLE JUICE	96
CHOCO LOVERS STRAWBERRY SHAKE	98
HEALTHY COFFEE SMOOTHIE	100
BLACKBERRY AND APPLE SMOOTHIE	102
LEMONY SPROUTS	103
COOL GARBANZO AND SPINACH BEANS	105

Fudge Brownies

Nutritional Facts

servings per container	9
Prep Total	**10 min**
Serving Size 2/3 cup (70g)	
Amount per serving **Calories**	10
	% Daily Value
Total Fat 20g	**2%**
Saturated Fat 2g	10%
Trans Fat 4g	-
Cholesterol	**10%**
Sodium 50mg	**12%**
Total Carbohydrate 7g	**20%**
Dietary Fiber 4g	7%
Total Sugar 12g	-
Protein 3g	
Vitamin C 2mcg	19%
Calcium 260mg	20%
Iron 8mg	8%
Potassium 235mg	6%

Ingredients

2 cups flour

2 cups of sugar

½ cup of cocoa powder

1 teaspoon baking powder

½ teaspoon salt

1 cup of vegetable oil

1 cup of water

1 teaspoon vanilla

1 cup dairy-free chocolate chips (optional)

½ cup chopped walnuts (optional)

Instructions:

1. Preheat oven to 350°F and grease a 9 x 13-inch baking pan.

2. Add dry ingredients in a mixing bowl. Whisk together wet ingredients and fold into the dry ingredients.

3. If desired, add half the chocolate chips and chopped walnuts to the mix. Pour mixture into the prepared pan and sprinkle with remaining chocolate chips and walnuts, if using.

4. For fudge-like brownies, bake for 20-25 minutes. For cake-like brownies, bake 25-30 minutes. Let the brownies cool slightly before serving.

Pomegranate Quinoa Porridge

Nutritional Facts

servings per container	4
Prep Total	10 min
Serving Size 2/3 cup (40g)	
Amount per serving **Calories**	22
	% Daily Value
Total Fat 12g	20%
Saturated Fat 2g	4%
Trans Fat 01g	1.22%
Cholesterol	22%
Sodium 170mg	10%
Total Carbohydrate 34g	22%
Dietary Fiber 5g	14%
Total Sugar 7g	-
Protein 3g	
Vitamin C 2mcg	10%
Calcium 260mg	20%
Iron 0mg	40%
Potassium 235mg	6%

Ingredients

1 1/2 cup quinoa flakes

2 1/2 teaspoons cinnamon

1 teaspoon vanilla extract

10 organic pDashes, pitted and cut into 1/4's

1 pomegranate pulp

1/4 cup desiccated coconut

Stewed apples

Coconut flakes to garnish

Instructions:

1. Gently place quinoa & almond milk into saucepan, & stir on medium to low heat for 9 minutes, until it smooth

2. Include cinnamon, desiccated coconut & vanilla extract & taste

3. Pit pDashes & cut into quarters include to porridge stir in well

4. Serve into individual bowls

5. Add a scoop of stewed apple (kindly view recipe below), pomegranates, pDashes & coconut flakes

Stewed apples

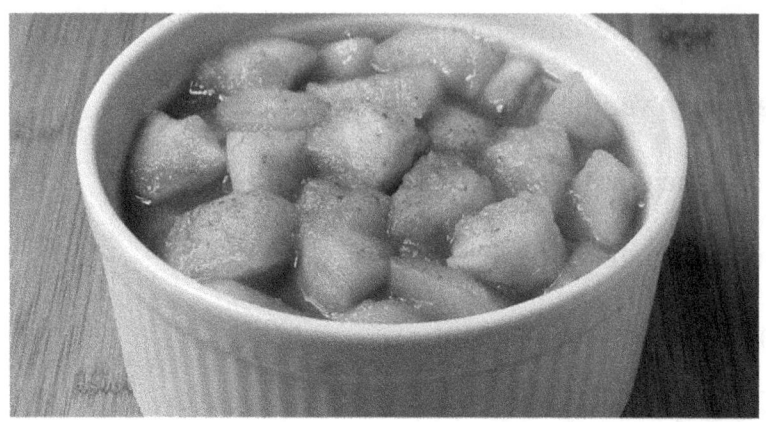

1. Peel, core, slice apples and place into a saucepan with water

2. Cook apples on medium heat, until extremely soft

3. Remove from heat, drain & mash apples

4. Ready to serve and enjoy your breakfast!

Cinnamon and Coconut Porridge

Serving: 4

Prep Time: 5 minutes

Cook Time: 5 minutes

Ingredients:

1 cup water

1/2 cup 36-percent low-fat cream

½ cup unsweetened dried coconut, shredded 1 tablespoon oat bran

1 tablespoon flaxseed meal

1/2 tablespoon almond butter

1 ½ teaspoons stevia

½ teaspoon cinnamon

Toppings, such as blueberries or banana slices

How To:

1. Add the ingredients to alittle pot and blend well until fully incorporated

2. Transfer the pot to your stove over medium-low heat and convey the combination to a slow boil.

3. Stir well and take away from the warmth .

4. Divide the mixture into equal servings and allow them to sit for 10 minutes.

5. Top together with your desired toppings and enjoy!

Nutrition (Per Serving)

Calories: 171

Fat: 16g

Protein: 2g

Carbohydrates: 8g

Coconut Porridge

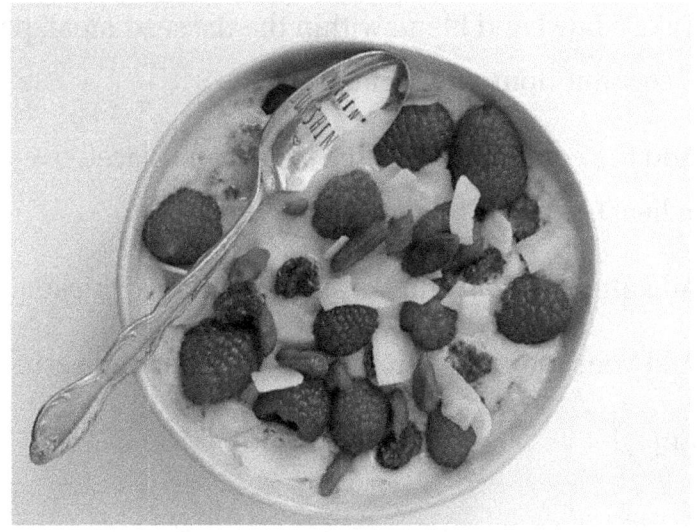

Serving: 2

Prep Time: 15 minutes

Cook Time: Nil

Ingredients:

2 tablespoons coconut flour

2 tablespoons vanilla protein powder

3 tablespoons Golden Flaxseed meal

1 ½ cups almond milk, unsweetened

Powdered Erythritol

How To:

1. Take a bowl and blend within the flaxseed meal, protein powder, coconut flour and blend well.

2. Add the combination to the saucepan (placed over medium heat).

3. Add almond milk and stir, let the mixture thicken.

4. Add your required amount of sweetener and serve.

5. Enjoy!

Nutrition (Per Serving)

Calories: 259

Fat: 13g

Carbohydrates: 5g

Protein: 16g

Cinnamon Pear Oatmeal

Serving: 2

Prep Time: 10 minutes

Cook Time: 15 minutes

Ingredients:

3 cups water

1 cup steel-cut oats

1 tablespoon cinnamon powder

1 cup pear, cored and peeled, cubed

How To:

1. Take a pot and add the water, oats, cinnamon, pear and toss well.

2. Bring it to simmer over medium heat.

3. Let it cook for quarter-hour , and divide into two bowls.

4. Enjoy!

Nutrition (Per Serving)

Calories: 171

Fat: 5g

Carbohydrates: 11g

Protein: 6g

Banana and Walnut Bowl

Serving: 4

Prep Time: 10 minutes

Cook Time: 15 minutes

Ingredients:

2 cups water

1 cup steel-cut oats

1 cup almond milk

¼ cup walnuts, chopped

2 tablespoons chia seeds

2 bananas, peeled and mashed

1 teaspoon vanilla flavoring

How To:

1. Take a pot and add all ingredients, toss well.
2. Bring it to simmer over medium heat.
3. Let it cook for quarter-hour , and divide into 4 bowls.

4. Enjoy!

Nutrition (Per Serving)

Calories: 162

Fat: 4g

Carbohydrates: 11g

Protein: 4g

Scrambled Pesto Eggs

Serving: 2

Prep Time: 5 minutes

Cook Time: 5 minutes

Ingredients:

2 large whole eggs

1/2 tablespoon almond butter

1/2 tablespoon pesto

1 tablespoon creamed coconut

almond milk

Sunflower seeds and pepper as needed

How To:

1. Take a bowl and crack open your eggs.
2. Season with a pinch of sunflower seeds and pepper.
3. Pour eggs into a pan.

4. Add almond butter and introduce heat.

5. Cook on low heat and gently add pesto.

6. Once the eggs are cooked and scrambled, remove from the warmth.

7. Spoon in coconut milk and blend well.

8. activate the warmth and cook on LOW for a short time until you've got a creamy texture.

9. Serve and enjoy!

Nutrition (Per Serving)

Calories: 467

Fat: 41g

Carbohydrates: 3g

Protein: 20g

Barley Porridge

Serving: 4

Prep Time: 5 minutes

Cook Time: 25 minutes

Ingredients:

1 cup barley

1 cup wheat berries

2 cups unsweetened almond milk

2 cups water

Toppings, such as hazelnuts, honey, berry, etc.

How To:

1. Take a medium saucepan and place it over medium-high heat.

2. Place barley, almond milk, wheat berries, water and convey to a boil.

3. Lower the warmth to low and simmer for 25 minutes.

4. Divide amongst serving bowls and top together with your desired toppings.

5. Serve and enjoy!

Nutrition (Per Serving)

Calories: 295

Fat: 8g

Carbohydrates: 56g

Protein: 6g

Mustard Chicken

Serving: 2

Prep Time: 10 minutes

Cook Time: 40 minutes

Ingredients:

2 chicken breasts

1/4 cup chicken broth

2 tablespoons mustard

1 1/2 tablespoons olive oil

1/2 teaspoon paprika

1/2 teaspoon chili powder

1/2 teaspoon garlic powder

How To:

1. Take alittle bowl and blend mustard, olive oil, paprika, chicken stock, garlic powder, chicken stock , and chili.

2. Add pigeon breast and marinate for half-hour .

3. Take a lined baking sheet and arrange the chicken.

4. Bake for 35 minutes at 375 degrees F.

5. Serve and enjoy!

Nutrition (Per Serving)

Calories: 531

Fat: 23g

Carbohydrates: 10g

Protein: 64g

Chicken and Carrot Stew

Serving: 4

Prep Time: 15 minutes

Cook Time: 6 hours

Ingredients:

4 boneless chicken breast, cubed

3 cups of carrots, peeled and cubed

1 cup onion, chopped

1 cup tomatoes, chopped

1 teaspoon of dried thyme

2 cups of chicken broth

2 garlic cloves, minced

Sunflower seeds and pepper as needed

How To:

1. Add all of the listed ingredients to a Slow Cooker.

2. Stir and shut the lid.

3. Cook for six hours.

4. Serve hot and enjoy!

Nutrition (Per Serving)

Calories: 182

Fat: 3g

Carbohydrates: 10g

Protein: 39g

The Delish Turkey Wrap

Serving: 6

Prep Time: 10 minutes

Cook Time: 10 minutes

Ingredients:

1 ¼ pounds ground turkey, lean

4 green onions, minced

1 tablespoon olive oil

1 garlic clove, minced

2 teaspoons chili paste

8-ounce water chestnut, diced

3 tablespoons hoisin sauce

2 tablespoon coconut aminos

1 tablespoon rice vinegar

12 almond butter lettuce leaves

1/8 teaspoon sunflower seeds

How To:

1. Take a pan and place it over medium heat, add turkey and garlic to the pan.

2. Heat for six minutes until cooked.

3. Take a bowl and transfer turkey to the bowl.

4. Add onions and water chestnuts.

5. Stir in duck sauce , coconut aminos, vinegar and chili paste.

6. Toss well and transfer mix to lettuce leaves.

7. Serve and enjoy!

Nutrition (Per Serving)

Calories: 162

Fat: 4g

Net Carbohydrates: 7g

Protein: 23g

Almond Butternut Chicken

Serving: 4

Prep Time: 15 minutes

Cook Time: 30 minutes

Ingredients:

½ pound Nitrate free bacon

6 chicken thighs, boneless and skinless

2-3 cups almond butternut squash, cubed Extra virgin olive oil Fresh chopped sage

Sunflower seeds and pepper as needed

How To:

1. Prepare your oven by preheating it to 425 degrees F.

2. Take an outsized skillet and place it over medium-high heat, add bacon and fry until crispy.

3. Take a slice of bacon and place it on the side, crumble the bacon.

4. Add cubed almond butternut squash within the bacon grease and sauté, season with sunflower seeds and pepper.

5. Once the squash is tender, remove skillet and transfer to a plate.

6. Add copra oil to the skillet and add chicken thighs, cook for 10 minutes.

7. Season with sunflower seeds and pepper.

8. Remove skillet from stove and transfer to oven.

9. Bake for 12-15 minutes, top with the crumbled bacon and sage.

10. Enjoy!

Nutrition (Per Serving)

Calories: 323

Fat: 19g

Carbohydrates: 8g

Protein: 12g

Zucchini Zoodles with Chicken and Basil

Serving: 3

Prep Time: 10 minutes

Cook Time: 10 minutes

Ingredients:

2 chicken fillets, cubed

2 tablespoons ghee

1-pound tomatoes, diced

½ cup basil, chopped

¼ cup almond milk

1 garlic clove, peeled, minced

1 zucchini, shredded

How To:

1. Sauté cubed chicken in ghee until not pink.
2. Add tomatoes and season with sunflower seeds.

3. Simmer and reduce liquid.

4. Prepare your zucchini Zoodles by shredding zucchini during a kitchen appliance .

5. Add basil, garlic, coconut almond milk to the chicken and cook for a couple of minutes.

6. Add half the zucchini Zoodles to a bowl and top with creamy tomato basil chicken.

7. Enjoy!

Nutrition (Per Serving)

Calories: 540

Fat: 27g

Carbohydrates: 13g

Protein: 59g

Beef Soup

Serving: 4

Prep Time: 10 minutes

Cook Time: 40 minutes

Ingredients:

1-pound ground beef, lean

1 cup mixed vegetables, frozen

1 yellow onion, chopped

6 cups vegetable broth

1 cup low-fat cream Pepper to taste

How To:

1. Take a stockpot and add all the ingredients the except cream, salt, and black pepper.

2. bring back a boil.

3. Reduce heat to simmer.

4. Cook for 40 minutes.

5. Once cooked, warm the cream .

6. Then add once the soup is cooked.

7. Blend the soup till smooth by using an immersion blender.

8. Season with salt and black pepper.

9. Serve and enjoy!

Nutrition (Per Serving)

Calories: 270

Fat: 14g

Carbohydrates: 6g

Protein: 29g

Amazing Grilled Chicken and Blueberry Salad

Serving: 5

Prep Time: 10 minutes

Cook Time: 25 minutes

Smart Points: 9

Ingredients:

5 cups mixed greens

1 cup blueberries

¼ cup slivered almonds

2 cups chicken breasts, cooked and cubed

For dressing

¼ cup olive oil

¼ cup apple cider vinegar

¼ cup blueberries

2 tablespoons honey

Sunflower seeds and pepper to taste

How To:

1. Take a bowl and add greens, berries, almonds, chicken cubes and blend well.

2. Take a bowl and blend the dressing ingredients, pour the combination into a blender and blitz until smooth.

3. Add dressing on top of the chicken cubes and toss well.

4. Season more and enjoy!

Nutrition (Per Serving)

Calories: 266

Fat: 17g

Carbohydrates: 18g

Protein: 10g

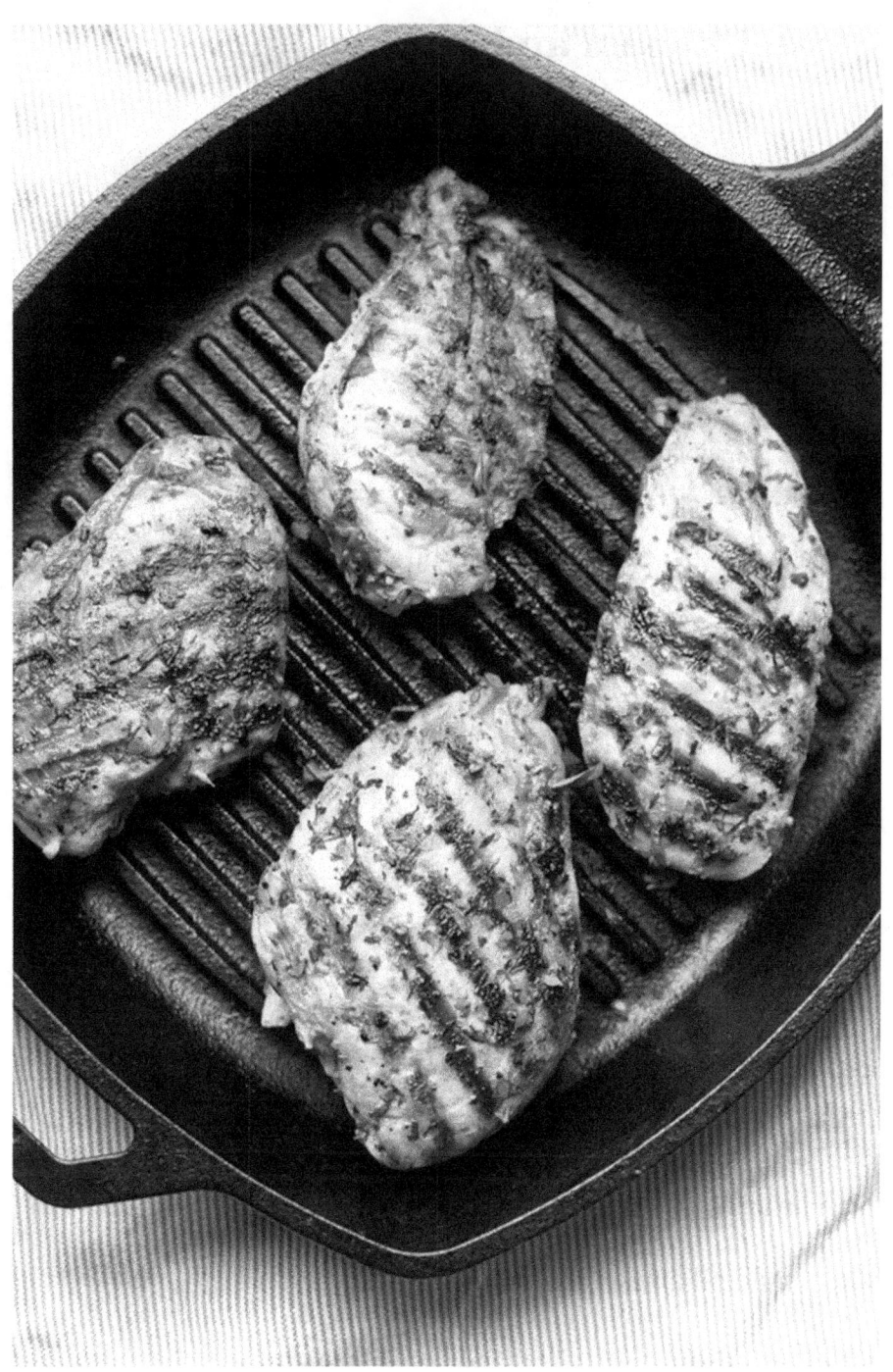

Clean Chicken and Mushroom Stew

Serving: 4

Prep Time: 10 minutes

Cook Time: 35 minutes

Ingredients:

4 chicken breast halves, cut into bite sized pieces

1 pound mushrooms, sliced (5-6 cups)

1 bunch spring onion, chopped

4 tablespoons olive oil

1 teaspoon thyme

Sunflower seeds and pepper as needed

How To:

1. Take an outsized deep frypan and place it over medium-high heat.

2. Add oil and let it heat up.

3. Add chicken and cook for 4-5 minutes per side until slightly browned.

4. Add spring onions and mushrooms, season with sunflower seeds and pepper consistent with your taste.

5. Stir.

6. Cover with lid and convey the combination to a boil.

7. Reduce heat and simmer for 25 minutes.

8. Serve!

Nutrition (Per Serving)

Calories: 247

Fat: 12g

Carbohydrates: 10g

Protein: 23g

Elegant Pumpkin Chili Dish

Serving: 4

Prep Time: 10 minutes

Cook Time: 15 minutes

Ingredients:

3 cups yellow onion, chopped

8 garlic cloves, chopped

1 pound turkey, ground

2 cans (15 ounces each) fire roasted tomatoes

2 cups pumpkin puree

1 cup chicken broth

4 teaspoons chili spice

1 teaspoon ground cinnamon

1 teaspoon sea sunflower seeds

How To:

1. Take an outsized sized pot and place it over medium-high heat.

2. Add copra oil and let the oil heat up.

3. Add onion and garlic, sauté for five minutes.

4. Add ground turkey and break it while cooking, cook for five minutes.

5. Add remaining ingredients and convey the combination to simmer.

6. Simmer for quarter-hour over low heat (lid off).

7. Pour chicken stock .

8. Serve with desired salad.

9. Enjoy!

Nutrition (Per Serving)

Calories: 312

Fat: 16g

Carbohydrates: 14g

Protein: 27g

Simple Garlic and Lemon Soup

Serving: 3

Prep Time: 10 minutes

Cook Time: nil

Ingredients:

1 avocado, pitted and chopped

1 cucumber, chopped

2 bunches spinach

1 ½ cups watermelon, chopped

1 bunch cilantro, roughly chopped

Juice from 2 lemons

½ cup coconut amines

½ cup lime juice

How To:

1. Add cucumber, avocado to your blender and pulse well.

2. Add cilantro, spinach and watermelon and blend.

3. Add lemon, juice and coconut amino.

4. Pulse a couple of more times.

5. Transfer to bowl and enjoy!

Nutrition (Per Serving)

Calories: 100

Fat: 7g

Carbohydrates: 6g

Protein: 3g

Healthy Cucumber Soup

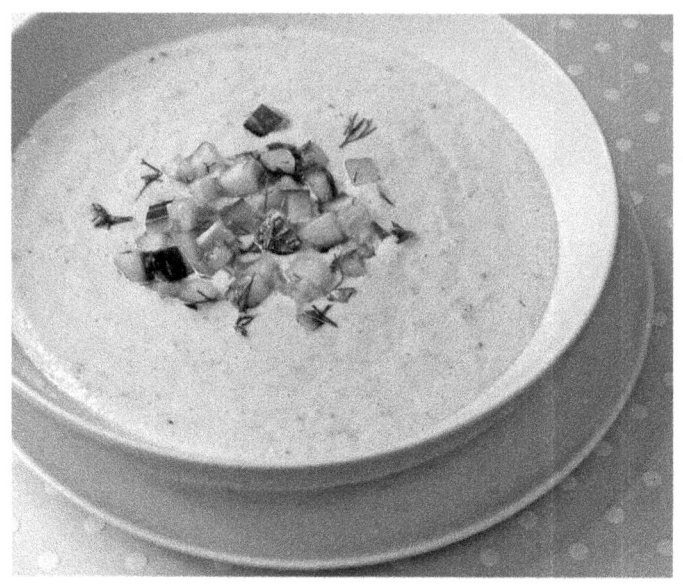

Serving: 4

Prep Time: 14 minutes

Cook Time: Nil

Ingredients:

2 tablespoons garlic, minced

4 cups English cucumbers, peeled and diced ½ cup onions, diced

1 tablespoon lemon juice 1 ½ cups vegetable broth ½ teaspoon sunflower seeds ¼ teaspoon red pepper flakes

¼ cup parsley, diced

½ cup Greek yogurt, plain

How To:

1. Add the listed ingredients to a blender and blend to emulsify (keep aside ½ cup of chopped cucumbers).

2. Blend until smooth.

3. Divide the soup amongst 4 servings and top with extra cucumbers.

4. Enjoy chilled!

Nutrition (Per Serving)

Calories: 371

Fat: 36g

Carbohydrates: 8g

Protein: 4g

Mushroom Cream Soup

Serving: 4

Prep Time: 5 minutes

Cook Time: 30 minutes

Ingredients:

1 tablespoon olive oil

½ large onion, diced

20 ounces mushrooms, sliced

6 garlic cloves, minced

2 cups vegetable broth

1 cup coconut cream

¾ teaspoon sunflower seeds

¼ teaspoon black pepper

1 cup almond milk

How To:

1. Take an outsized sized pot and place it over medium heat.

2. Add onion and mushrooms to the vegetable oil and sauté for 10-15 minutes.

3. confirm to stay stirring it from time to time until browned evenly.

4. Add garlic and sauté for 10 minutes more.

5. Add vegetable broth, coconut milk , almond milk[MOU6], black pepper and sunflower seeds.

6. Bring it to a boil and lower the temperature to low.

7. Simmer for quarter-hour .

8. Use an immersion blender to puree the mixture.

9. Enjoy!

Nutrition (Per Serving)

Calories: 200

Fat: 17g

Carbohydrates: 5g

Protein: 4g

Curious Roasted Garlic Soup

Serving: 10

Prep Time: 10 minutes

Cook Time: 60 minutes

Ingredients:

1 tablespoon olive oil

2 bulbs garlic, peeled

3 shallots, chopped

1 large head cauliflower, chopped

6 cups vegetable broth

Sunflower seeds and pepper to taste

How To:

1. Pre-heat your oven to 400 degrees F.

2. Slice ¼ inch top of garlic bulb and place it in aluminum foil.

3. Grease with vegetable oil and roast in oven for 35 minutes.

4. Squeeze flesh out of the roasted garlic.

5. Heat oil in saucepan and add shallots, sauté for six minutes.

6. Add garlic and remaining ingredients.

7. Cover pan and reduce heat to low.

8. Let it cook for 15-20 minutes.

9. Use an immersion blender to puree the mixture. 10. Season soup with sunflower seeds and pepper.

10. Serve and enjoy!

Nutrition (Per Serving)

Calories: 142

Fat: 8g

Carbohydrates: 3.4g

Protein: 4g

Amazing Roasted Carrot Soup

Serving: 4

Prep Time: 10 minutes

Cook Time: 50 minutes

Ingredients:

8 large carrots, washed and peeled

6 tablespoons olive oil

1-quart broth

Cayenne pepper to taste

Sunflower seeds and pepper to taste

How To:

1. Pre-heat your oven to 425 degrees F.

2. Take a baking sheet and add carrots, drizzle vegetable oil and roast for 30-45 minutes.

3. Put roasted carrots into blender and add broth, puree.

4. Pour into saucepan and warmth soup.

5. Season with sunflower seeds, pepper and cayenne.

6. Drizzle vegetable oil .

7. Serve and enjoy!

Nutrition (Per Serving)

Calories: 222

Fat: 18g

Net Carbohydrates: 7g

Protein: 5g

Simple Pumpkin Soup

Serving: 4

Prep Time: 5 minutes

Cook Time: 6-8 hours

Ingredients:

1 small pumpkin, halved, peeled, seeds removed, cubed

2 cups chicken broth

1 cup coconut milk

Pepper and thyme to taste

How To:

1. Add all the ingredients to a crockpot.
2. Close the lid.
3. Cook for 6-8 hours on low.
4. Make a smooth puree by employing a blender.
5. Garnish with roasted seeds.

6. Serve and enjoy!

Nutrition (Per Serving)

Calories: 60

Fat: 2g

Net Carbohydrates: 10g

Protein: 3g

Coconut Avocado Soup

Serving: 4

Prep Time: 5 minutes

Cook Time: 5-10 minutes

Ingredients:

2 cups vegetable stock

2 teaspoons Thai green curry paste

Pepper as needed

1 avocado, chopped

1 tablespoon cilantro, chopped

Lime wedges

1 cup coconut milk

How To:

1. Add milk, avocado, curry paste, pepper to blender and blend.

2. Take a pan and place it over medium heat.

3. Add mixture and warmth, simmer for five minutes.

4. Stir in seasoning, cilantro and simmer for 1 minute.

5. Serve and enjoy!

Nutrition (Per Serving)

Calories: 250

Fat: 30g

Net Carbohydrates: 2g

Protein: 4g

Coconut Arugula Soup

Serving: 4

Prep Time: 5 minutes

Cook Time: 5-10 minutes

Ingredients:

Black pepper as needed

1 tablespoon olive oil

2 tablespoons chives, chopped

2 garlic cloves, minced

10 ounces baby arugula

2 tablespoons tarragon, chopped

4 tablespoons coconut milk yogurt

6 cups chicken stock

2 tablespoons mint, chopped

1 onion, chopped

½ cup coconut milk

How To:

1. Take a saucepan and place it over medium-high heat, add oil and let it heat up.

2. Add onion and garlic and fry for five minutes.

3. Stir available and reduce the warmth, let it simmer.

4. Stir in tarragon, arugula, mint, parsley and cook for six minutes.

5. Mix in seasoning, chives, coconut yogurt and serve.

6. Enjoy!

Nutrition (Per Serving)

Calories: 180

Fat: 14g

Net Carbohydrates: 20g

Protein: 2g

Awesome Cabbage Soup

Serving: 3

Prep Time: 7 minutes

Cook Time: 25 minutes

Ingredients:

3 cups non-fat beef stock

2 garlic cloves, minced

1 tablespoon tomato paste

2 cups cabbage, chopped

½ yellow onion

½ cup carrot, chopped

½ cup green beans

½ cup zucchini, chopped

½ teaspoon basil

½ teaspoon oregano

Sunflower seeds and pepper as needed

How To:

1. Grease a pot with non-stick cooking spray.

2. Place it over medium heat and permit the oil to heat up.

3. Add onions, carrots, and garlic and sauté for five minutes.

4. Add broth, ingredient, green beans, cabbage, basil, oregano, sunflower seeds, and pepper.

5. Bring the entire mix to a boil and reduce the warmth, simmer for 5-10 minutes until all veggies are tender.

6. Add zucchini and simmer for five minutes more.

7. Sever hot and enjoy!

Nutrition (Per Serving)

Calories: 22

Fat: 0g

Carbohydrates: 5g

Protein: 1g

Baked Zucchini Wrapped Fish

Serving: 2

Prep Time: 15 minutes

Cook Time: 15 minutes

Ingredients:

24-ounce cod fillets, skin removed

tablespoon of blackening spices

zucchini, sliced lengthwise to form ribbon

½ tablespoon of olive oil

How To:

1. Season the fish fillets with blackening spice.
2. Wrap each fillet with zucchini ribbons.
3. Place fish on a plate.
4. Take a skillet and place over medium heat.
5. Pour oil and permit the oil to heat up.

6. Add wrapped fish to the skillet and cook all sides for 4 minutes.

7. Serve and enjoy!

Nutrition (Per Serving)

Calories: 397

Fat: 23g

Carbohydrates: 2g

Protein: 46g

Heart-Warming Medi Tilapia

Serving: 4

Prep Time: 15 minutes

Cook Time: 15 minutes

Ingredients:

tablespoons sun-dried tomatoes, packed in oil, drained and chopped

tablespoon capers, drained

tilapia fillets

tablespoon oil from sun-dried tomatoes tablespoons kalamata olives, chopped and pitted

How To:

1. Pre-heat your oven to 372 degrees F.

2. Take alittle sized bowl and add sun-dried tomatoes, olives, capers and stir well.

3. Keep the mixture on the side.

4. Take a baking sheet and transfer the tilapia fillets and arrange them side by side.

5. Drizzle vegetable oil everywhere them.

6. Bake in your oven for 10-15 minutes.

7. After 10 minutes, check the fish for a "Flaky" texture.

8. Once cooked, top the fish with the tomato mixture and serve!

Nutrition (Per Serving)

Calories: 183

Fat: 8g

Carbohydrates: 18g

Protein:83g

Baked Salmon and Orange Juice

Serving: 2

Prep Time: 10 minutes

Cook Time: 10 minutes

Ingredients:

½ pound salmon steak

Juice of 1 orange

Pinch ginger powder, black pepper, and sunflower seeds

Juice of ½ lemon

1-ounce coconut almond milk

How To:

1. Preheat oven to 350 degrees F.

2. Rub salmon steak with spices and let it sit for quarter-hour.

3. Take a bowl and squeeze an orange.

4. Squeeze juice also and blend.

5. Pour almond milk into the mixture and stir.

6. Take a baking dish and line with aluminium foil .

7. Place steak thereon and pour the sauce over steak.

8. Cover with another sheet and bake for 10 minutes.

9. Serve and enjoy!

Nutrition (Per Serving)

Calories: 300

Fat: 3g

Carbohydrates: 1g

Protein: 7g

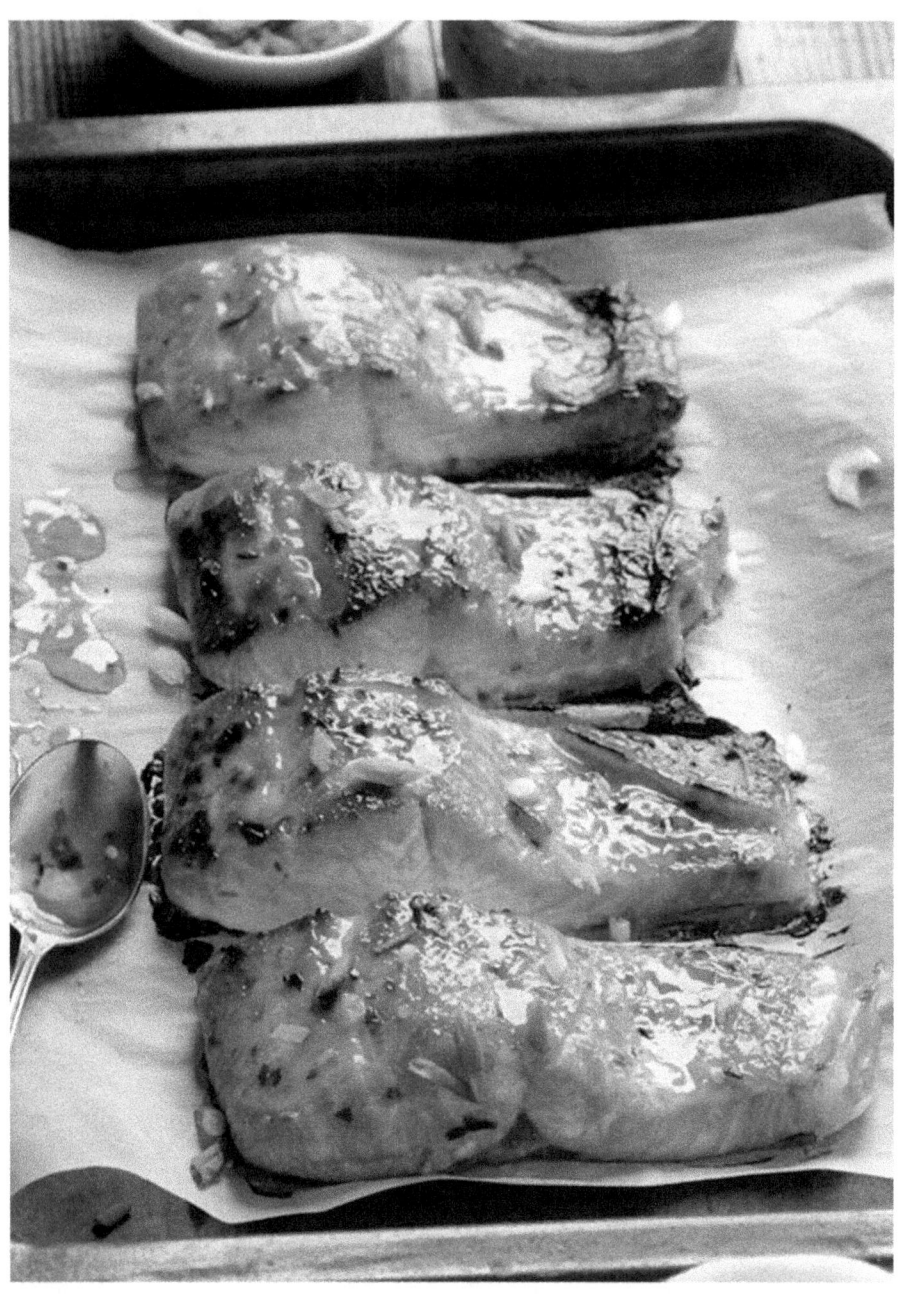

Lemon and Almond butter Cod

Serving: 2

Prep Time: 5 minutes

Cook Time: 20 minutes

Ingredients:

tablespoons almond butter, divided thyme sprigs, fresh and divided teaspoons lemon juice, fresh and divided

cod fillets, 6 ounces each Sunflower seeds to taste

How To:

1. Pre-heat your oven to 400 degrees F.

2. Season cod fillets with sunflower seeds on each side.

3. Take four pieces of foil, each foil should be 3 times bigger than the fillets.

4. Divide fillets between the foil and top with almond butter, juice, thyme.

5. Fold to make a pouch and transfer pouches to the baking sheet.

6. Bake for 20 minutes.

7. Open and let the steam out.

8. Serve and enjoy!

Nutrition (Per Serving)

Calories: 284

Fat: 18g

Carbohydrates: 2g

Protein: 32g

Shrimp Scampi

Serving: 4

Prep Time: 25 minutes

Cook Time: Nil

Ingredients:

teaspoons olive oil

1 ¼ pounds medium shrimp

6-8 garlic cloves, minced

½ cup low sodium chicken broth

½ cup dry white wine

¼ cup fresh lemon juice

¼ cup fresh parsley + 1 tablespoon extra, minced ¼ teaspoon sunflower seeds

¼ teaspoon fresh ground pepper

slices lemon

How To:

1. Take an outsized sized bowl and place it over medium-high heat.

2. Add oil and permit the oil to heat up.

3. Add shrimp and cook for 2-3 minutes.

4. Add garlic and cook for 30 seconds.

5. Take a slotted spoon and transfer the cooked shrimp to a serving platter.

6. Add broth, juice, wine, ¼ cup of parsley, pepper, and sunflower seeds to the skillet.

7. Bring the entire mix to a boil.

8. Keep boiling until the sauce has been reduced to half.

9. Spoon the sauce over the cooked shrimp.

10. Garnish with parsley and lemon.

11. Serve and enjoy!

Nutrition (Per Serving)

Calories: 184
Fat: 6g
Carbohydrates: 6g
Protein: 15g

Light Beef Chili

SmartPoints value: Green plan - 4SP, Blue plan - 4SP, Purple plan – 4SP

Total Time: 2hrs 30mins, Prep time: 30mins, Cooking time: 2hrs, Serves: 8

Nutritional value: Calories - 187, Carbs – 24g, Fat – 3g, Protein – 16g

This red meat dish is perfect for warming up on a chilly day. One of the reasons I love it is because preparing it is very easy. Often, I will make this chili, then measure and place each of them in a Ziploc bag and refrigerate. Whenever I need something hot and filling, all I need to do is grab one and microwave.

Ingredients

Beef bouillon powder - 1 tbsp

Bell pepper (red, diced) - 1 small

Black pepper - 1/2 tsp

Brewed coffee (strong) - 1 cup

Chili powder - 3 tbsp

Cocoa (unsweetened) - 1 tsp

Cumin - 2 tbsp

Dark beer - One 12oz can

Garlic (minced) - 4 cloves

Green pepper (diced) - 1 small

Ground beef (extra lean) - 1 lb

Kidney beans - One 15oz can

Onion (diced) - 1 large

Oregano - 2 tsp

Paprika - 1 tsp

Salt - 1 tsp

Sugar - 1 tbsp

Tomatoes (diced) - One 28oz can

Tomato sauce - One 8oz can

Instructions

1. Place a large pot or Dutch oven over medium-high heat and spray it with non-fat cooking spray.

2. Add the onions and garlic, then cook until onions start to soften; about 3 minutes.

3. Toss in the ground beef and cook until the meat turns brown.

4. Add the diced bell peppers to the beef and cook for another 5 minutes.

5. Put in all the remaining ingredients asides the kidney beans and stir.

6. Bring the content of the pot to a simmer, then stir in the kidney beans.

7. Reduce the heat to medium-low, cover the pot, and let it cook for about 2 hours.

This perfect hearty beef chili made with extra lean ground beef simmers in fantastic spices and flavors to give you a desirable taste.

Insalata Greca

Nutrition

Calories: 326 kcal | Gross carbohydrates: 11 g | Protein: 14 g | Fats: 26 g |

Fiber: 4 g | Net carbohydrates: 7 g | Macro fats: 55 % | Macro proteins: 30 % |

Macro carbohydrates: 15 %

Total time: 5 minutes

Ingredients

50 grams of tomato

50 grams of cucumber

25 grams of red pepper or yellow pepper

15 grams of red onion

50 grams of feta

50 grams of black olives

3 tablespoons extra virgin olive oil

1 tablespoon lemon juice

1 teaspoon dried oregano

1 egg

Instructions

1. Bring a saucepan of water to the boil. Once the water boils, place the egg in it. Boil the egg for 8 minutes.

2. Clean the onion and cut into thin slices (keep the rest of the onion in a sealed container in the refrigerator).

3. Wash the tomato, pepper, and cucumber and cut the pepper and cucumber into thin slices. Dice the tomato.

4. Peel the egg and cut it into slices.

5. Arrange the tomatoes and the egg in the center of a plate. Put the cucumber slices around it. Place the bell pepper and red onion on top of the tomatoes.

6. Drain the feta if necessary and cut into small 1 cm large cubes. Place in a heap on top of the tomato.

7. Decorate the dish with the black olives and sprinkle the oregano over the tomatoes.

8. Make the vinaigrette in a small cup or bowl by mixing the olive oil and lemon juice well with a fork or teaspoon.

9. Pour the vinaigrette over the salad.

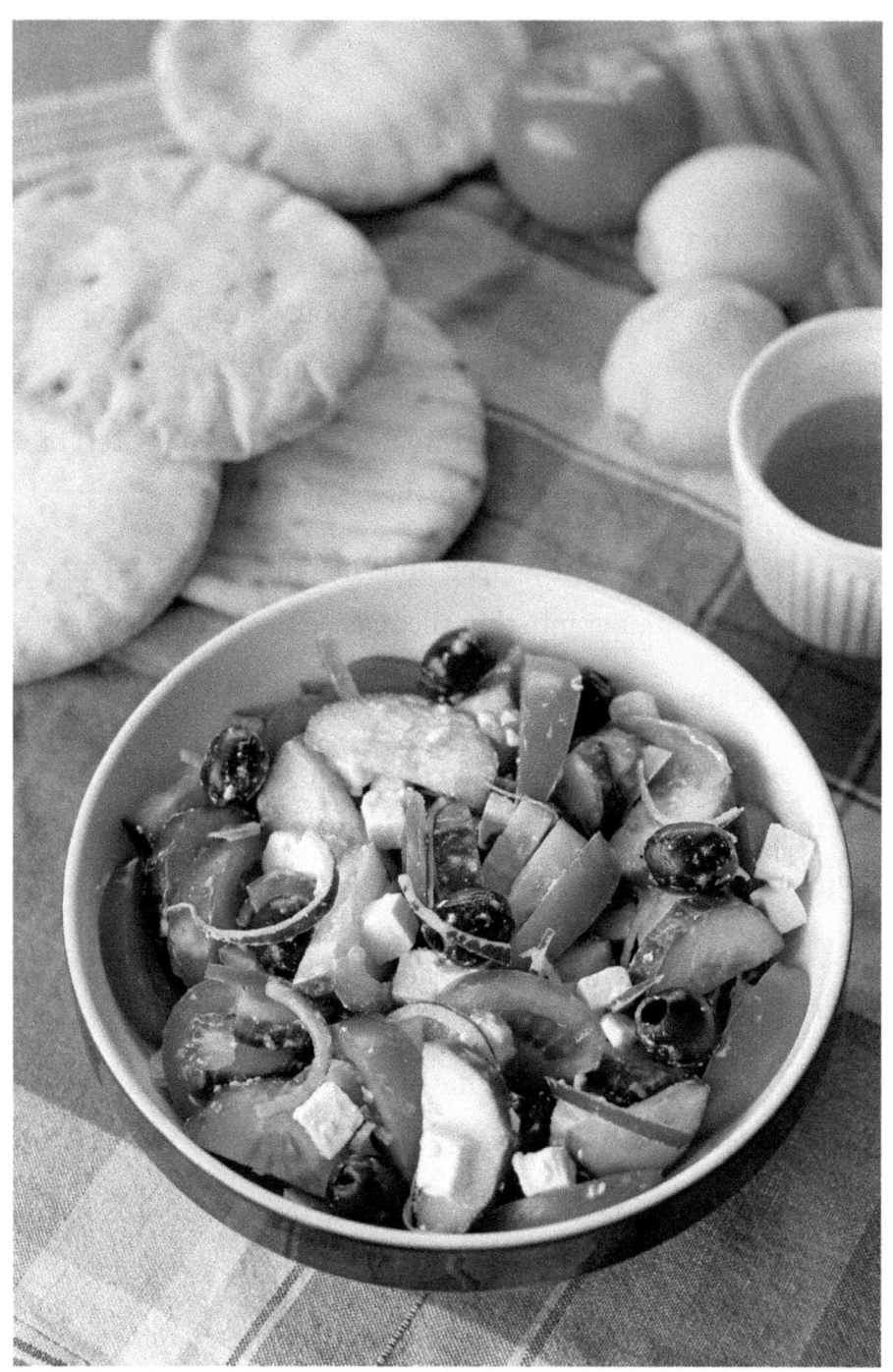

Crudities

Nutrition

Calories: 22 kcal | Gross carbohydrates: 5 g | Protein: 1 g | Fats: 0.2 g | Fiber: 2 g | Net carbohydrates: 3 g | Macro fat: 5 % | Macro proteins: 24 % | Macro carbohydrates: 71 %

Total time: 10 minutes

Ingredients

1 celery stem

1 bush of chicory cuts lengthwise into four pieces Cut 10 cm cucumber into long, thin strips

2 peppers, for example, red and yellow

Instructions

1. Cut the vegetables into thin, long strips so that you can dip them. For example, you can use chicory, little gem lettuce, cucumber, colored peppers, and celery.

2. Tasty and fast - if you don't feel like cooking.

Herring with Onions

Nutrition

Calories: 111 kcal | Gross carbohydrates: 3 g | Protein: 12 g | Fats: 6 g | Fiber:0.3 g | Net carbohydrates: 3 g | Macro fat: 29 % | Macro proteins: 58 % |Macro carbohydrates: 13 %

Time - 15 minutes

Ingredients

1 haring

1 tablespoon onion

Instructions

A very quick lunch.

Notes

If you follow the keto diet, you can still get some goodies from the fish stall.

Tasty and very healthy! Herring contains many Omega 3 fatty acids.

Simple Gingerbread Muffins

Serving: 12

Prep Time: 5 minutes

Cooking Time: 30 minutes

Ingredients:

1 tablespoon ground flaxseed

6 tablespoons coconut almond milk

1 tablespoon apple cider vinegar

½ cup peanut almond butter

2 tablespoons gingerbread spice blend

1 teaspoon baking powder

1 teaspoon vanilla extract

2 tablespoons Swerve

How To:

1. Pre-heat your oven to 350 degrees F.

2. Take a bowl and add flaxseeds, sweetener, sunflower seeds, vanilla, spices and your non-dairy almond milk.

3. Keep it on the side for a while.

4. Add peanut almond butter, baking powder and keep mixing until combined well.

5. Stir in peanut almond butter and baking powder.

6. Mix well.

7. Spoon the mixture into muffin liners.

8. Bake for 30 minutes.

9. Allow them to cool and enjoy!

Nutrition (Per Serving)

Total Carbs: 13g

Fiber: 4g

Protein: 11g

Fat: 23g

Fantastic Cauliflower Bagels

Serving: 12

Prep Time: 10 minutes

Cooking Time: 30 minutes

Ingredients:

1 large cauliflower, divided into florets and roughly chopped

¼ cup nutritional yeast

¼ cup almond flour

½ teaspoon garlic powder

1 ½ teaspoon fine sea sunflower seeds

1 whole egg

1 tablespoon sesame seeds

How To:

1. Pre-heat your oven to 400 degrees F.

2. Line a baking sheet with parchment paper, keep it on the side.

3. Blend cauliflower in the food processor and transfer to a bowl.

4. Add nutritional yeast, almond flour, garlic powder and sunflower seeds to a bowl, mix.

5. Take another bowl and whisk in eggs, add to cauliflower mix.

6. Give the dough a stir.

7. Incorporate the mix into the egg mix.

8. Make balls from dough, making a hole using your thumb into each ball.

9. Arrange them on your prepped sheet, flattening them into bagel shapes.

10. Sprinkle sesame seeds and bake for 30 minutes.

11. Remove oven and let them cool, enjoy!

Nutrition (Per Serving)

Total Carbs: 1.5g

Fiber: 1g

Protein: 2g

Fat: 5.8g

Nutmeg Nougats

Serving: 12

Prep Time: 10 minutes

Cooking Time: 5 minutes

Freeze Time: 30 minutes

Ingredients:

1 cup coconut, shredded

1 cup low-fat cream

1 cup cashew almond butter

½ teaspoon ground nutmeg

How To:

1. Melt the cashew almond butter over a double boiler.
2. Stir in nutmeg and dairy cream.
3. Remove from the heat.
4. Allow to cool down a little.

5. Keep in the refrigerator for at least 30 minutes.

6. Take out from the fridge and make small balls.

7. Coat with shredded coconut.

8. Let it cool for 2 hours and then serve.

Nutrition (Per Serving)

Total Carbs: 13g

Fiber: 8g

Protein: 3g

Fat: 34g

Limey Savory Pie

Serving: 12

Prep Time: 5 minutes

Cooking Time: 5 minutes

Freeze Time: 2 hours

Ingredients:

1 tablespoon ground cinnamon

3 tablespoons almond butter

1 cup almond flour

For the filling:

3 tablespoons grass-fed almond butter

4 ounces full-fat cream cheese

¼ cup coconut oil

2 limes

A handful of baby spinach Stevia to taste

How To:

1. Mix cinnamon and almond butter to form a crumble mixture.

2. Press this mixture into the bottom of 12 muffin cups.

3. Bake for 7 minutes at 350 degrees F.

4. Juice the lime and grate for zest while the crust is baking.

5. Take a food processor and add all the filling ingredients.

6. Blend until smooth.

7. Let it cool naturally.

8. Pour the mixture in the center.

9. Freeze until set and serve.

Nutrition (Per Serving)

Total Carbs: 2g

Fiber: 1g

Protein: 3g

Fat: 1g

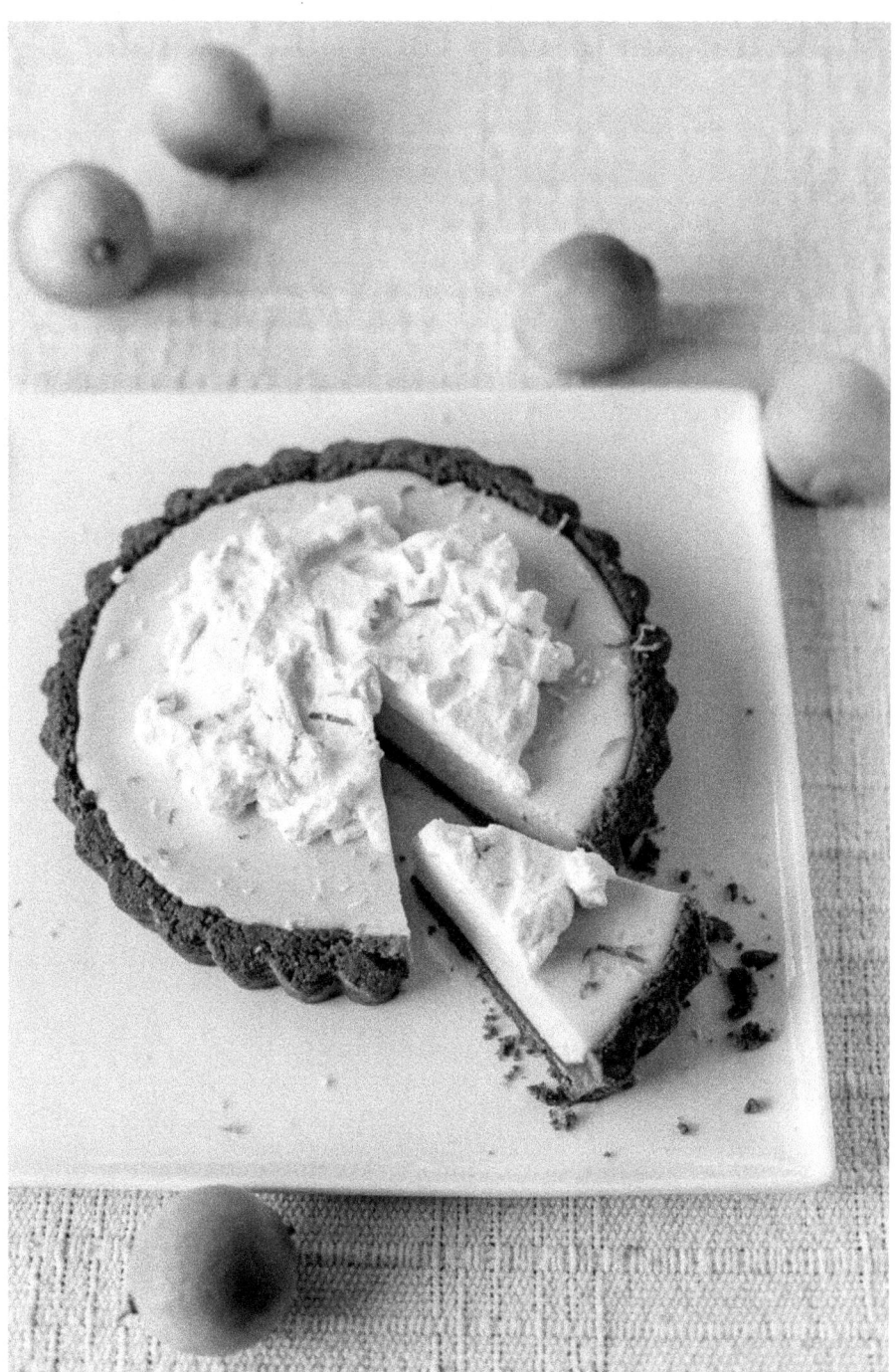

Supreme Raspberry Chocolate Bombs

Serving: 6

Prep Time: 10 minutes

Cooking Time: 10 minutes

Freeze Time: 1-hour

Ingredients:

½ cacao almond butter

½ coconut manna

4 tablespoons powdered coconut almond milk

3 tablespoons granulated stevia

¼ cup dried and crushed raspberries, frozen

How To:

1. Prepare your double boiler to medium heat and melt the cacao almond butter and coconut manna.

2. Stir in vanilla extract.

3. Take another dish and add coconut powder and sugar substitute.

4. Stir the coconut mix into the cacao almond butter, 1 tablespoon at a time, making sure to keep mixing after each addition.

5. Add the crushed dried raspberries.

6. Mix well and portion it out into muffin tins.

7. Chill for 60 minutes and enjoy!

Nutrition (Per Serving)

Total Carbs: 7g

Fiber: 1g

Protein: 11g

Fat: 21g

The Perfect Orange Ponzu

Serving: 8

Prep Time: 30 minutes

Cook Time: 5 minutes

Ingredients:

¼ cup coconut aminos

½ cup rice vinegar

2 tablespoons dry fish flakes

1 (1 inch) square kombu (kelp)

1 orange, quartered

How To:

1. Take a saucepan and place it over medium heat.

2. Add coconut aminos, rice vinegar, fish flakes, kombu, orange quarters and let the mixture sit for 30 minutes.

3. Bring the mix to a boil and immediately remove from the heat.

4. Let it cool and strain through a cheesecloth.

5. Serve and enjoy!

Nutrition (Per Serving)

Calories: 15

Fat: 0g

Carbohydrates: 4g

Protein: 0.8g

Hearty Cashew and Almond butter

Serving: 1 and ½ cups

Prep Time: 5 minutes

Cook Time: Nil

Ingredients:

1 cup almonds, blanched

1/3 cup cashew nuts

2 tablespoons coconut oil

Sunflower seeds as needed

½ teaspoon cinnamon

How To:

1. Pre-heat your oven to 350 degrees F.
2. Bake almonds and cashews for 12 minutes.
3. Let them cool.
4. Transfer to food processor and add remaining ingredients.

5. Add oil and keep blending until smooth.

6. Serve and enjoy!

Nutrition (Per Serving)

Calories: 205

Fat: 19g

Carbohydrates: g[MOU3]

Protein: 2.8g

Refreshing Mango and Pear Smoothie

Serving: 1

Prep Time: 10 minutes

Cook Time: Nil

Ingredients:

1 ripe mango, cored and chopped

½ mango, peeled, pitted and chopped

1 cup kale, chopped

½ cup plain Greek yogurt

2 ice cubes

How To:

1. Add pear, mango, yogurt, kale, and mango to a blender and puree.

2. Add ice and blend until you have a smooth texture.

3. Serve and enjoy!

Nutrition (Per Serving)

Calories: 293

Fat: 8g

Carbohydrates: 53g

Protein: 8g

Epic Pineapple Juice

Serving: 4

Prep Time: 10 minutes

Cook Time: nil

Ingredients:

4 cups fresh pineapple, chopped

1 pinch sunflower seeds

1 ½ cups water

How To:

1. Add the listed ingredients to your blender and blend well until you have a smoothie-like texture.

2. Chill and serve.

3. Enjoy!

Nutrition (Per Serving)

Calories: 82

Fat: 0.2g

Carbohydrates: 21g

Protein: 21

Choco Lovers Strawberry Shake

Serving: 1

Prep Time: 10 minutes

Ingredients:

½ cup heavy cream, liquid

1 tablespoon cocoa powder

1 pack stevia

½ cup strawberry, sliced

1 tablespoon coconut flakes, unsweetened

1 ½ cups water

How To:

1. Add listed ingredients to blender.
2. Blend until you have a smooth and creamy texture.
3. Serve chilled and enjoy!

Nutrition (Per Serving)

Calories: 470

Fat: 46g

Carbohydrates: 15g

Protein: 4g

Healthy Coffee Smoothie

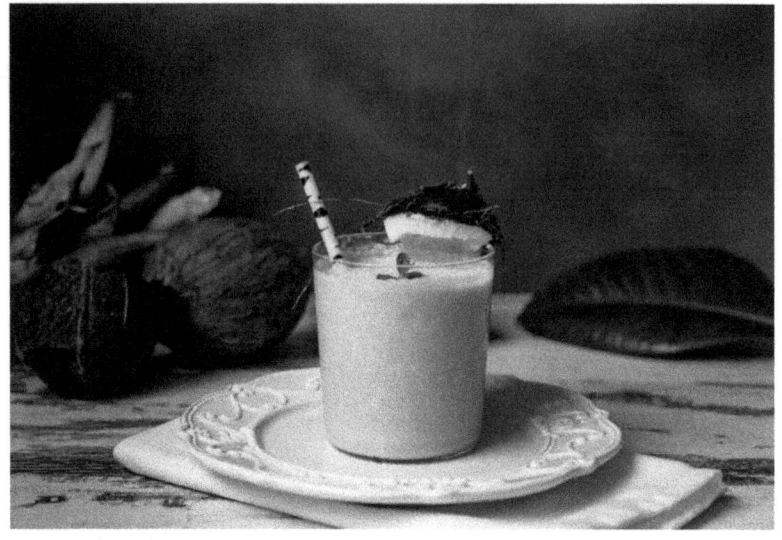

Serving: 1

Prep Time: 10 minutes

Ingredients:

1 tablespoon chia seeds

2 cups strongly brewed coffee, chilled

1-ounce Macadamia Nuts

1-2 packets stevia, optional

1 tablespoon MCT oil

How To:

1. Add all the listed ingredients to a blender.

2. Blend on high until smooth and creamy.

3. Enjoy your smoothie.

Nutrition (Per Serving)

Calories: 395

Fat: 39g

Carbohydrates: 11g

Protein: 5.2g

Blackberry and Apple Smoothie

Serving: 2

Prep Time: 5 minutes

Ingredients:

2 cups frozen blackberries

½ cup apple cider

1 apple, cubed

2/3 cup non-fat lemon yogurt

How To:

1. Add the listed ingredients to your blender and blend until smooth.
2. Serve chilled!

Nutrition (Per Serving)

Calories: 200
Fat: 10g
Carbohydrates: 14g
Protein 2g

Lemony Sprouts

Serving: 4

Prep Time: 10 minutes

Cook Time: Nil

Ingredients:

1 pound Brussels sprouts, trimmed and shredded

8 tablespoons olive oil

1 lemon, juice and zested

Sunflower seeds and pepper to taste

¾ cup spicy almond and seed mix

How To:

1. Take a bowl and mix in lemon juice, sunflower seeds, pepper and olive oil.
2. Mix well.
3. Stir in shredded Brussels sprouts and toss.
4. Let it sit for 10 minutes.
5. Add nuts and toss.
6. Serve and enjoy!

Nutrition (Per Serving)

Calories: 382

Fat: 36g

Carbohydrates: 9g

Protein: 7g

Cool Garbanzo and Spinach Beans

Serving: 4

Prep Time: 5-10 minutes

Cook Time: Nil

Ingredients:

1 tablespoon olive oil

½ onion, diced

10 ounces spinach, chopped

12 ounces garbanzo beans

½ teaspoon cumin

How To:

1. Take a skillet and add olive oil, let it warm over medium-low heat.

2. Add onions, garbanzo and cook for 5 minutes.

3. Stir in spinach, cumin, garbanzo beans and season with sunflower seeds.

4. Use a spoon to smash gently.

5. Cook thoroughly until heated, enjoy!

Nutrition (Per Serving)

Calories: 90

Fat: 4g

Carbohydrates:11g

Protein:4g

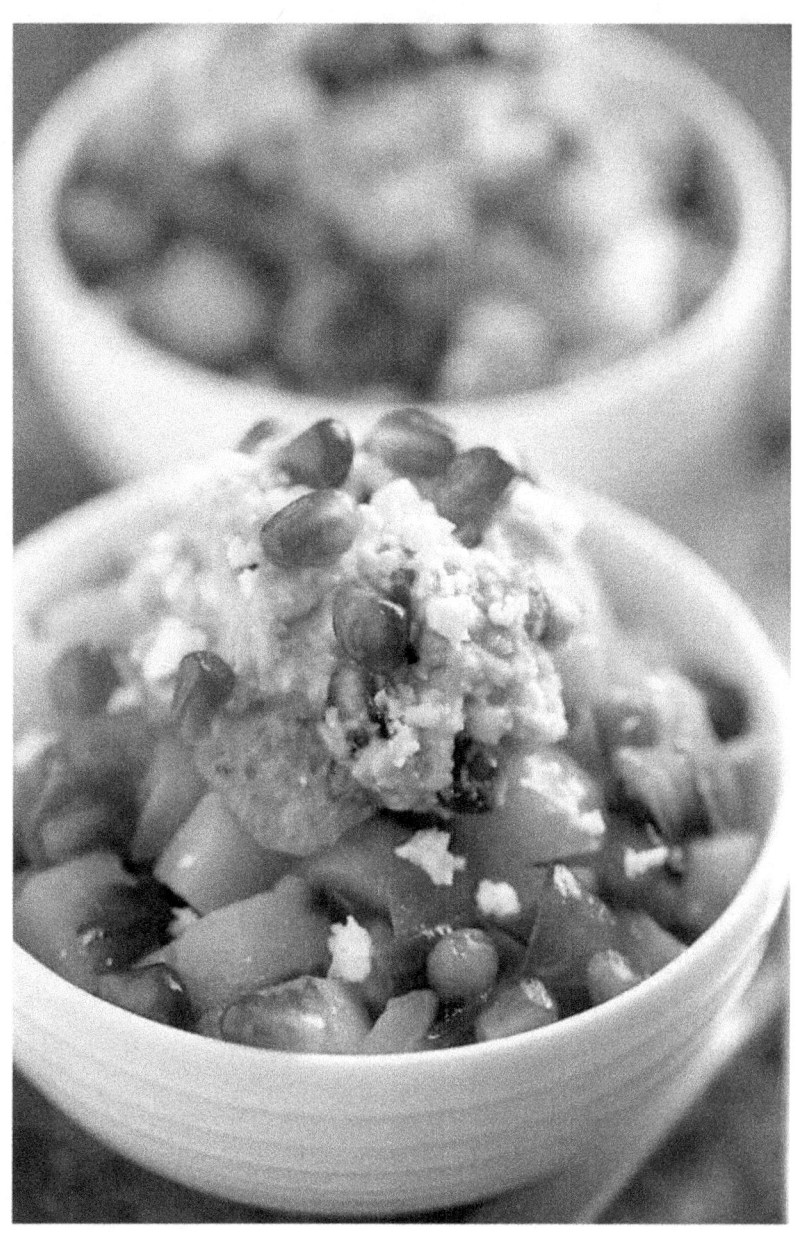

www.ingramcontent.com/pod-product-compliance
Lightning Source LLC
Chambersburg PA
CBHW071111030426
42336CB00013BA/2034